Frequently Asked Questions

all about
B vitamins

BURT BERKSON MD, PhD

AVERY PUBLISHING GROUP
Garden City Park • New York

The information contained in this book is based upon the research and personal and professional experiences of the author. They are not intended as a substitute for consulting with your physician or other health care provider. Any attempt to diagnose and treat an illness should be done under the direction of a health care professional.

The publisher does not advocate the use of any particular health care protocol, but believes the information in this book should be available to the public. The publisher and author are not responsible for any adverse effects or consequences resulting from the use of any of the suggestions, preparations, or procedures discussed in this book. Should the reader have any questions concerning the appropriateness of any procedure or preparation mentioned, the author and the publisher strongly suggest consulting a professional health care advisor.

Series cover designer: Eric Macaluso
Cover image courtesy of Barry Axelrod Studios, Inc.

ISBN: 0-89529-908-9

Printed in the United States of America

10   9   8   7   6   5   4   3   2   1

Contents

Introduction, 5

1. The Amazing B Vitamins, 9
2. Vitamin B_1 (Thiamin), 19
3. Vitamin B_2 (Riboflavin), 29
4. Vitamin B_3 (Niacin and Niacinamide), 35
5. Pantothenic Acid, 43
6. Vitamin B_6 and Folic Acid, 49
7. Vitamin B_{12}, 63
8. Choline and Inositol, 71
9. Biotin and PABA, 81

Conclusion, 87

Glossary, 89

References, 91

Suggested Readings, 93

Index, 95

Introduction

Ronald Hartman, a 45-year-old attorney in New York City, was having trouble concentrating on his work. He passed some time watching an attractive co-worker from down the hall through the glass wall of his office and began to feel impulsive. He knew her name was Robin, and he had seen her at the Downtown Athletic Club almost every day after work. He decided he wanted to know her better.

That evening, at the health club, Ronald walked up to Robin as she was doing sit-ups on the incline board. When she finished, he started chatting. He said that he had worked late that evening and was going out to dinner alone. He asked her to join him and she agreed. After showering and dressing, they got into his car and drove uptown where they had a delicious dinner of prime rib with grilled spring mushrooms.

Later in the evening, as they were riding the elevator up to Robin's apartment, Ronald experienced severe nausea. He asked to use her bathroom and began to vomit. Soon afterwards, Robin suffered similar symptoms. It wasn't the greatest first date. The two of them drove up to New York Hospital's emergency room.

The ER physician asked if they ate anything unusual for dinner, and they told him about the spring mushrooms. He immediately called the Center for Disease Control in Atlanta, and they gave him my name and telephone number. The doctor called me at my home and explained the situation to me. I asked him to check the source of the mushrooms. He did and soon called me back. The mushrooms were an imported hand-picked variety from Asia. I realized that the mushroom picker must have inadvertently gathered some poisonous mushrooms along with the harmless morels (spring mushrooms). I suggested that the doctor start an intravenous infusion of a vitamin B_6, also known as pyridoxine, solution for the two patients. He did—and they survived.

Why did a simple vitamin save the lives of these two people? The mushroom toxin in this case depleted the patient's storehouse of vitamin B_6, a nutrient essential for the body's production of proteins and infection-fighting antibodies. It is also necessary for the production of the stomach acid that starts the process of food digestion and for the production of the nucleic acids that form genes.

Ronald Hartman was thankful for the life-saving powers of this common B vitamin. However, when his wife in a New Jersey suburb found out that he was in a New York hospital with an equally impaired dinner date, she decided to file for divorce. This is a true story. I have only changed the names of the characters and their location.

The B vitamins may not prevent divorce, but they do many other things besides protect you from death by poisonous mushrooms. During one week in my office, I used B vitamins to treat heart disease, high cholesterol, poor immune function, headaches, anemia, genital herpes, and shingles. The B vitamins work together as a team and support the health of the skin, the nervous system, the brain, the eyes, digestive tract, and the internal organs. Some B vitamins are substances that stimulate the enzymes that produce energy, and others may alleviate schizophrenia. Pyridoxine, folic acid, and cobalamin—various B vitamins—may prevent heart attacks and strokes by cleaning up high levels of a substance called homocysteine, which can cause cardiovascular diseases. Other B vitamins can elevate your mood naturally. Doctors that understand vitamin therapy—orthomolecular doctors—realize that this therapy should involve tailored doses and various combinations of B vitamins.

You have certainly heard of the B vitamins. They

include thiamin (B_1), riboflavin (B_2), niacin (B_3), pantothenic acid (B_5), pyridoxine (B_6), cobalamin (B_{12}), folic acid, biotin, choline, inositol, and para-aminobenzoic acid (PABA). They have different functions and have very distinct chemical structures. You need them all in the correct amounts and in the proper balance to continue living a healthy life. By reading *All About B Vitamins*, you'll discover the importance of these vital substances and the impact that they have on your health.

Before you read any further, I do have some guidance in terms of taking B vitamins and their dosages. When people are deficient, they are rarely deficient in just one B vitamin. In addition, the B vitamins work best as a family of nutrients. Keeping these thoughts in mind, as a general rule, it's important to always take a B-complex supplement when taking extra amounts of any single B vitamin. (Of course, if your physician advises otherwise, follow his instructions.) For example, if you take folic acid and vitamin B_{12}, round out your supplementation regimen with a complete B-complex supplement. Doing so will promote the natural synergism of all the B vitamins. I believe that most people will benefit from a B-complex supplement (or the equivalent as part of a multivitamin supplement). Your health-food store or pharmacy can provide you with further guidance in selecting a specific product.

1.

The Amazing B Vitamins

In this chapter, I provide a general overview of the B-complex vitamins, describe some of their functions, and answer some general questions about them. In other chapters, I'll go into more detail about what each of the B vitamins does and how they can benefit your health. Perhaps the most important point to remember is that the B vitamins may not have the publicity pizzazz of antioxidants, but that they are extremely important to your physical health and mental well being.

Q. What exactly are the B vitamins?

A. There are several distinct nutrients recognized as B-complex vitamins. They are all water-soluble, indispensable for a multitude of bodily functions, and often work together as a team. Some B vitamins cannot be adequately stored in the body, so you must consume them daily. Others can be stored. If you are on a strict weight-loss diet, eat a lot of processed food, frequently take antibiotics or seizure disorder drugs, drink a substantial amount of alcohol, or are inclined to fast, you may be deficient in one or more of the B vitamins.

Vitamins, by definition, are nutrients that cannot be made by your body. This definition does not always hold true because some of the B vitamins are produced in small amounts in your digestive tract or in your organs. The vitamins were given letter designations because of their long technical names. It's easier to use the term vitamin B_6 instead of the word pyridoxine.

Q. Why do I need the B-complex vitamins?

A. You require this group of nutrients for the well-being of your blood and immune systems, the transformation of food into usable energy, proper nervous system function, good heart health, and for many other purposes that will be discussed further along in this book.

Q. In what foods can I find the B vitamins?

A. The B vitamins are found in many kinds of foods. They are often naturally grouped together in various combinations in order to help one another do their jobs. The organ meats, such as liver or kidney, are excellent sources of B-complex vitamins. Muscle meats, such as T-bone steaks, are not very high in this group, but do contain high levels of vitamin B_{12}.

If you are a vegetarian, whole grains, legumes (such as beans and peas), and leafy green vegetables are good sources of B-complex vitamins. Over the last 100 years, people have preferred that the food manufacturers produce a cereal product that looks clean, so it is stripped of its bran and germ. These products are almost devoid of B-complex vitamins. You won't find natural B-complex vitamins in white bread, most pasta, breakfast cereals, and the like. Most manufacturers today add some artificial B vitamins to their product.

Q. Do the RDAs provide adequate levels of B vitamins?

A. I do not believe that the RDAs provide adequate levels of B vitamins. The RDAs were instituted during World War II—more than 50 years ago— to alleviate dangerous vitamin deficiency diseases, such as pellagra (B_3 deficiency) and beriberi (B_1 deficiency). These suggestions were only the minimum doses required to prevent these flagrant deficiency syndromes. The signs and symptoms of vitamin deficiencies are more elusive than the gross symptoms of vitamin deficiency diseases. Fatigue, pins and needles in your toes, pale color, painful tongue, and numerous other symptoms may be warning you that you are heading for a serious vitamin deficiency. In my opinion, most adults could benefit from taking about three times the RDA, and often even more, of the B vitamins.

Q. Do antibiotics deplete my B-vitamin levels?

A. Yes, they do. Beneficial bacteria that normally live in your large intestines can manufacture very small amounts of some B vitamins. If you are taking certain antibiotics, the helpful bacteria may be killed, and you may become vitamin deficient. It is important to replace your intestinal bacteria during and after antibiotic use with an acidophilus (good bacteria) supplement. You should continue taking the bacterial preparation for 2 weeks after stopping the antibiotic.

Q. I cook most of my food. Can heat destroy the B vitamins?

A. Cooking or microwaving food may destroy the potency of several B vitamins. As we grow older, it is more important to get additional B-complex vitamins to stay healthy. If you do cook your food, it would be a good idea to supplement your diet with B-complex capsules. Also, try to eat more raw foods, such as leafy green salads.

Q. Why are so many Americans deficient in B-complex vitamins?

A. This is because so many of us eat a diet that is very low in or devoid of B-complex vitamins. For example, large amounts of simple sugars, refined flour bakery goods, and fast foods are sometimes devoid of B-complex vitamins. Companies that produce these products often add one artificial B vitamin or another, but in my opinion, this is not acceptable for your good health. Stick with the whole grains, beans, and other natural products, and stay away from the highly processed foods.

Q. Can the B-complex vitamins protect me from heart disease?

A. Yes, they can. Many physicians and researchers believe that an elevated homocysteine level is an important risk factor for serious damage to the arteries and subsequent heart disease. Homocysteine is a byproduct produced during the breakdown of protein. In one of many studies, scientists have reported that supplementation with B-complex vitamins significantly lowered the homocysteine serum levels in over 600 individuals. The key B vitamins in this respect are folic acid and vitamin B_6. The minimal dose for reducing homocysteine levels and cardiovascular risk is about 400 mcg of folic acid and 7 mg of vitamin B_6.

Q. Do some of the B vitamins have antioxidant properties?

A. Yes. Pantothenic acid and vitamin B_6, in the proper doses, have the ability to act as antioxidants—free radical scavengers—and protect against the destruction of cell membranes and the mutation of DNA by free radicals.

Q. Can B-complex vitamins protect a person from cancer?

A. Yes, I believe the B vitamins play important roles in preventing cancer. Most cancers start with a mutation, or a random change, to deoxyribonucleic acid (DNA), which forms genes and chromosomes. A lack of folic acid (a B vitamin) interferes with DNA's ability to repair damage. In one recent study, conducted in Australia, researchers found that high supplemental amounts of folic acid and vitamin B_{12} lowered levels of chromosome damage in otherwise healthy young adults. The accumulation of such damage is one of the basic causes of aging and cancer.

Q. Can B-complex vitamins improve my mood and reduce stress?

A. The B vitamins have a long history as "antistress" nutrients and mood enhancers. This should not be entirely surprising because B-complex vitamins are necessary for healthy brain function. Several scientists have suggested that the initial signs of B-vitamin insufficiency are irritability and difficulty in dealing with stress. Psychological studies have found that providing students with high-potency vitamins made them more agreeable and improved their moods.

Q. What should be my daily dose of B vitamins?

A. I think that doses of vitamins should be specifically tailored for each person depending on his or her diet, sex, body weight, age, occupation, condition of health, and the amount of exercise they perform each day. Personally, I take a daily high-quality B-complex capsule twice a day that includes 25 mg B_1, 25 mg B_2, 25 mg niacin (B_3), 125 mg niacinamide (B_3), 150 mg pantothenic acid, 50 mg B_6, 400 mcg B_{12}, 800 mcg folic acid, 400 mcg biotin, 50 mg choline, 50 mg inositol, and 50 mg PABA. When I feel I might be developing a virus, I double this dose.

You may need less or more. One of my friends used to take a regular B-complex supplement, but he had dandruff. One day he heard that some of the B vitamins might help in eczema. He figured that these were both skin disorders, so he started taking a higher potency B-complex supplement. This was more than 25 years ago. His dandruff cleared in a few days and has never returned.

Q. Can B-complex vitamins be toxic?

A. Any substance in extremely high doses, even water and B vitamins, can be toxic. In addition, because of the interrelated jobs of the B vitamins, they should be taken as B complex. If you take too much of one B vitamin for too long, you may suppress the activity of another B vitamin and that may cause a deficiency. If you feel you need to take high doses of a single B vitamins, you should take a B-complex supplement for additional nutritional support.

2.

Vitamin B$_1$ (Thiamin)

Vitamin B$_1$, also known as thiamin, is usually found as a large and complicated molecule called thiamin pyrophosphate in humans and other animals. This vitamin is important because it is part of the biochemical series of reactions that release stored energy from foods. Thiamin also helps in the synthesis of the chemicals that pass messages from one nerve cell to another, called neurotransmitters. You should obtain thiamin in your diet every day; however, small amounts of it are stored in your liver and kidneys. Excess thiamin is eliminated in your urine and perspiration.

Q. What foods must I eat to get proper amounts of thiamin?

A. Thiamin is found in relatively high concentrations in whole grains that have all of their parts intact. In America, we usually encounter these grains with the important parts removed, such as in white bread and pastas. The good parts of whole grains are removed mechanically and fed to farm animals because it makes them healthy. You will get high levels of thiamin if you eat whole cereal grains, egg yolks, fresh beans, fish, brewer's yeast supplements, and pork.

Q. What does beriberi have to do with vitamin B_1?

A. Beriberi is the name given to a severe deficiency of vitamin B_1. This deficiency disease is characterized by diarrhea, edema, fatigue, and weight loss. Severe symptoms can lead to heart failure and nerve damage that can cause paralysis.

Beriberi became noticeable during World War II in prisoners of war in Asia who were given refined rice that had been mechanically stripped of the outer, nutrient-rich shell. In 1997, a study was published describing a number of other disease conditions found in concentration camps that might be associated with thiamin deficiency. Among these conditions were salivary gland cysts, inguinal hernias, and carpal tunnel syndrome. It appears that thiamin, in addition to its other roles, functions to help hold your connective tissue together.

Q. What exactly does thiamin do for my health?

A. Thiamin is a coenzyme that helps the body's biochemical catalysts (enzymes) to do their jobs. Through this action, thiamin is necessary for carbohydrate metabolism, normal digestion, and the formation of your blood. It is also needed to break down alcohol into its harmless end products, carbon dioxide and water.

In addition, thiamin is indispensable for the proper function of your adrenal glands. These endocrine structures produce hormones that manage various types of mental, immunological, and physical stress. Animals that lack thiamin often develop adrenal tumors and suppressed immune systems, making them susceptible to infections.

Thiamin is also required for the production of acetylcholine, an important chemical that passes messages from one nerve to another. And, among other important roles, thiamin, with the help of other substances such as lipoic acid, may reduce the formation of plaque in the arteries that supply the heart with blood.

Q. How can I tell if I am thiamin deficient?

A. A severely thiamin deficient person first notices fatigue, poor memory, abdominal pains, and constipation. This condition may continue to progress to palpitations of your heart, pins and needles in your feet, muscle weakness, and vision problems. If you have these symptoms, you should see a doctor; if they are the result of vitamin deficiency, supplementation should be prescribed.

Q. I am a smoker. How can thiamin help me?

A. Smoking causes a build up of the toxic products of oxidation in your tissues. Bedsides acting as a coenzyme, thiamin functions as an antioxidant, scavenging these oxidation byproducts. Consequently, it can help protect you to some extent from the toxic garbage that results from excess alcohol consumption and smoking.

Q. Can eating a lot of junk foods cause symptoms of thiamin deficiency?

A. Yes, I think so. Soft drinks, French fries, numerous desserts, and other unhealthy fast foods have been linked to thiamin deficiency, along with acne and nervous problems.

Q. Will drinking too much alcohol cause thiamin deficiency?

A. Many cases of thiamin deficiency are caused by alcoholism. Such a deficiency reduces the breakdown of simple sugars and creates a decrease in the utilization of oxygen and results in poor brain function. People who drink excessive amounts of alcohol on a regular basis also often have poor dietary thiamin intake, diminished thiamin absorption, and decreased thiamin storage. If they continue to drink immoderately, they could develop beriberi-type heart disease, permanent neurological damage, and die.

Q. I've been told that thiamin can modify certain genetic diseases. Is that really true?

A. Yes. Some biologists have always understood that genes are not necessarily "written in stone." And nutrients have been shown to modify the expression of specific genes. For example, both aspirin and butyrate (a byproduct of dietary fiber) modify genes that are necessary for the growth of colon cancer.

Thiamin is another example of a common molecule that changes the way a gene is expressed, or gets turned on. Certain children have one virus infection after another. Their lymph nodes are always enlarged, and they have low-grade fevers. This condition is caused by an inherited abnormal gene and can lead to an early death. Derrick Lonsdale, MD, of Cleveland, has treated such children with relatively high doses of thiamin, and their symptoms have disappeared. When the thiamin supplementation was stopped, the symptoms came back. Dr. Lonsdale found that just by giving the sick children some thiamin, he was able to make them healthy again.

Q. How much thiamin should I take each day?

A. Of course, vitamin dosages must be tailored for each individual, and it's best to take the entire B complex. The Recommended Daily Allowance (RDA) for thiamin is very low—1.5 mg daily for an adult. I take at least 50–100 mg of thiamin every day. That's quite a difference, of course, but I think it is the difference between barely preventing beriberi and achieving some measure of optimal health. Many people have told me that by increasing their thiamin intake, along with a balance of other vitamins, they feel an enormous increase in energy.

Q. Is it true that thiamin can improve disposition?

A. Dr. David Benton of the University of Wales, Swansea, administered thiamin to a group of college volunteers who had symptoms of depression. He found that they became more clear-headed, energetic, and self-composed after only three months of treatment. Nutritionally oriented doctors often use thiamin with a balance of other supplements to treat chronic fatigue, depression, and lack of self-esteem. The dosage range of thiamin for this use tends to be 50–100 mg daily. Once again, take a B-complex supplement along with higher dosages of B_1. Alternatively, consider taking a high-potency B-complex that already has 50 mg of B_1.

Q. Can thiamin supplementation make me smarter?

A. It won't give you the mind of Albert Einstein, but it might make you a little sharper. When a group from the United Kingdom wanted to determine the long-term impact of vitamin supplementation on over 120 adults, they found that enhanced thiamin status improved performance on a wide range of cognitive function tests in women, but not in men. So, my answer is, conditionally, yes.

Q. Can thiamin help in cases of Bell's palsy?

A. Bell's palsy is a paralysis of the facial nerve. It often develops as a result of injury to the nerve or some emotional stress. I think it is a viral infection of the facial nerve, and I regularly use a variety of B vitamins for this condition, especially thiamin and pantothenic acid. I have also had good luck using it to treat another painful facial condition called trigeminal neuralgia.

Q. Do people need more thiamin as they get older?

A. Generally yes. Scientists find that about 50 percent of nursing home patients have low thiamin levels. In Belgium, doctors reported that geriatric patients had only about 50 percent of the amount of thiamin in the brain as found in infants. It might even help in Alzheimer's disease. A group of researchers in Toronto, Canada reported that thiamin supplementation provided modest improvement of brain function in Alzheimer's patients.

Q. Some people with diabetes take thiamin to alleviate diabetic neuropathies. How would this work?

A. Diabetic neuropathies start out as a hypersensitivity to light touch. When this condition is in advanced stages, it causes burning pains in the extremities, especially the feet, and disables the diabetic patient. The actual neuropathy (nerve damage) is related to the high blood sugar levels and related injuries to the blood vessels feeding the nerves.

Many doctors only suppress the pain with drugs. Other doctors treat the cause of diabetes, rather than just relieving symptoms. They put their patients on strict but sensible diets and prescribe vitamins, antioxidants, and a reasonable exercise program. The use of thiamin, along with another amazing supplement alpha-lipoic acid, encourages the blood vessels and nerves of the skin to utilize sugar more efficiently. With this type of natural treatment, many of my patients become free of the pain.

3.

Vitamin B$_2$ (Riboflavin)

Vitamin B$_2$, or riboflavin, is a distinctively yellow molecule and vitamin. It is more resistant to heat than thiamin, so it does not break down as easily during cooking. It is, however, very sensitive to light, so foods and supplements containing it should be protected from sunlight. Riboflavin is a fundamental component of a molecule called flavin adenine dinucleotide (FAD), which is needed for energy production in your body.

Q. Is there a disease condition caused by a vitamin B$_2$ deficiency?

A. This condition is called "ariboflavinosis." Patients with this fairly common condition show up at the doctor's office with weakness, sore throat, crusty material at the corners of their mouths, painful mouths, red and sore tongues, and eye problems. At times they suffer a type of anemia associated with poor red cell production in the bone marrow.

Q. What are the best sources of riboflavin?

A. The organ meats, such as liver, kidney, and pancreas, are especially high in this vitamin. Probably even better sources of riboflavin are certain algae and brewer's yeast.

Q. What are some common causes of riboflavin deficiency?

A. One recent medical journal article reported that male smokers had lower levels of riboflavin than nonsmokers. In addition, extremely low-fat diets in teenagers may result in lower vitamin status and possibly deficiencies in riboflavin and other important nutrients. In general, a poor diet and deficiencies of other nutrients may signal a possible deficiency of vitamin B_2.

Q. Can additional riboflavin cure migraine headaches?

A. Yes, in certain cases. Doctors may prescribe a short course of 400 mg per day of riboflavin to patients with migraines. They often see improvement in over half of the patients. In one double-blind research study, high doses of riboflavin significantly decreased the frequency of headaches in eighty migraine patients over a period of one year. It's not likely that riboflavin will reverse migraines, but it should be very helpful in preventing them.

Q. Can low riboflavin levels contribute to the development of cancer?

A. Yes. In a recent study, animals were fed cancer-causing chemicals that resulted in gene mutations. These mutations were self-repaired by animals with high riboflavin levels, but were not repaired by riboflavin-deficient animals. It is quite possible that riboflavin has a place in the prevention of cancer in people.

Q. Can riboflavin help with rheumatoid arthritis?

A. People with this condition feel much worse when they are under oxidative stress—that is when they are exposed to too many hazardous molecules called free radicals. So it is important to ingest the proper amount of antioxidants, such as vitamins E and C, to ease this problem. Scientists have reported that riboflavin supplements, which have antioxidant activity, may help people with rheumatoid arthritis feel better.

Q. My urine turns yellow from riboflavin—is this dangerous?

A. It is not dangerous at all. Riboflavin crystals have a yellow fluorescent glow. The color is the result of excess riboflavin being excreted in the urine. This means that your body has used the amount that it needs and has excreted the rest, it does not mean that the riboflavin is not being absorbed.

Q. Why is riboflavin necessary for life?

A. Riboflavin, like thiamin, is necessary for the operation of certain chemical cycles that produce energy. Riboflavin is needed for the construction of at least two fundamental coenzymes that carry energy to the high-energy storage molecule ATP. Your cells could not effectively utilize oxygen without riboflavin. Consequently, riboflavin is required for the life of your cells.

Q. Is crusty stuff at the corners of the mouth related to riboflavin deficiency?

A. Yes, crusty material at the corners of the mouth is characteristic of riboflavin deficiency and is medically called cheilosis. A shortage of other B vitamin can also cause this condition.

Q. How much riboflavin should I take?

A. In general, I think most people would benefit from 10 to 25 mg of riboflavin as part of a B-complex supplement. If you think you are deficient in this vitamin, or feel you need more, discuss your situation with a health professional.

4.

Vitamin B$_3$ (Niacin and Niacinamide)

Vitamin B$_3$ is available as a supplement in two forms: niacin (nicotinic acid) and niacinamide (nicotinamide). Like vitamins B$_1$ and B$_2$, it is also required for the production of energy in the body. One of the major discoveries related to vitamin B$_3$ is that it can improve some types of schizophrenia, particularly recent schizophrenia. The niacin, but not niacinamide, form of B$_3$ can also lower cholesterol levels. In this chapter, when I refer to vitamin B$_3$, I mean either niacin or niacinamide. Please be aware that niacin causes a body-wide tingling and flushing sensation, which decreases with regular use of the supplement.

Q. What is the RDA for vitamin B$_3$, and what foods contain it?

A. The RDA for vitamin B$_3$ is about 15 to 20 mg. I

take at least 50 mg of niacin and 250 mg of niacinamide each day as a maintenance dose. The foods
that contain the greatest amounts of niacin are the
high-protein foods, such as organ meats. Whole-
grain cereals and legumes such as peanuts and
beans also contain high levels of niacin.

Q. Do doctors ever use vitamin B_3 to treat diseases?

A. Yes, high niacin doses effectively reduce bad
cholesterol levels called low-density lipoproteins
(LDL) and raise good cholesterol levels called high-
density lipoproteins (HDL). Numerous studies
have shown that niacin works as well as prescription drugs, but without the dangerous side effects.
As a cholesterol-lowering agent, 200 to 500 mg of
niacin, taken three times daily, should be helpful.
The main side effect that most people notice is a
harmless body-wide tingling sensation and flushing of the skin. This reaction diminishes with regular use of the supplement. Julian Whitaker, MD, a
well-known physician, recommends a form of
niacin called inositol hexanicotinate because it does
not seem to cause skin flushing. The niacinamide
form of B_3 does not cause flushing, but it does not
lower cholesterol either.

A form of cholesterol called "lipoprotein (a)" is

an important risk factor in coronary heart disease. Niacin and vitamin C reduce lipoprotein (a) levels by decreasing its production in the liver.

Some psychiatrists and neurologists use niacin and niacinamide to treat serious mental and neurological diseases, such as schizophrenia, epilepsy, and Parkinson's disease. Abram Hoffer, MD, PhD, of Victoria, Canada, pioneered the use of vitamin B_3 in the treatment of schizophrenia. Both niacin and niacinamide are effective for this disorder. For schizophrenia, Hoffer tends to start patients on 3 g (3,000 mg) of niacin or niacinamide, plus 3 g of vitamin C daily. This is a relatively high dose, and patients should have their liver enzymes checked by a physician. While generally safe, high doses of niacin or niacinamide sometimes cause liver problems.

Another blood vessel problem that niacin can be used to treat is a painful condition called Raynaud's syndrome. Often, people with autoimmune diseases such as scleroderma and lupus develop episodes of aching fingertips when exposed to various conditions such as cold temperatures. This is due to constriction of blood vessels in the fingertips and the accumulation of antibodies in these regions. This condition often leads to sloughing off of the tissues of the fingers, including the nails, and serious infections. High doses of niacin can help this problem by increasing blood flow to the fingers.

Q. I've heard that low levels of niacin might predispose a person to cancer—is this true?

A. It might. A number of researchers believe that a vitamin B_3 deficiency could lead to a shortage of nicotinamide adenine dinucleotide (NAD), a molecule that carries energy in cells. People with cancers often have low levels of NAD. I think that a better understanding of niacin metabolism may lead to a better comprehension of cancer prevention.

One group of scientists fed animals B_3-deficient diets and found that all of them developed cancer. This is because vitamin B_3 is required for the repair of broken strands of genes. There have been many other studies that show that niacin can repair DNA damage in human white blood cells and thereby assist the proficiency of the immune system.

Vitamin B_3 is also necessary for the synthesis of coenzyme Q_{10}, a vitamin-like substance, and there is evidence that it may be a therapy for some forms of cancer. I would think that vitamin B_3 in the proper doses would protect you from some forms of malignant disease.

Q. Can vitamin B₃ lower aggressive tendencies?

A. Possibly yes. Scientists have found that vitamin B_3 supplementation decreases aggressive behavior in male animals. They hypothesize that niacin increases serotonin levels, creating a feeling of well-being. Many antidepressant drugs and the antidepressant herb St. John's wort also raise serotonin levels.

Q. What are the early signs and symptoms of a niacin deficiency?

A. Just as with other specific B vitamin deficiencies, the first manifestations are weakness, sore mouth and tongue, weight loss, and nervous irritability.

Q. How can a doctor diagnose pellagra?

A. Advanced pellagra can be diagnosed by medical tests. The breakdown products of niacin are found in people who suffer from pellagra. Also, low blood levels of NAD may show that a person is sick with pellagra. The symptoms include dermatitis, diarrhea, and dementia.

Q. Don't some people with advanced AIDS develop pellagra-like symptoms?

A. There has not been a great amount of research in this particular field. Many doctors who treat AIDS prescribe niacin supplements, and some researchers have demonstrated that in dishes of cells, niacinamide can inhibit the growth of the virus that causes AIDS. Patients with AIDS typically have multiple vitamin and mineral deficiencies, and RDA levels will not restore normal levels. Higher doses are required.

Q. Is niacin ever toxic?

A. The niacin flush can be very frightening if you don't expect it, but it is not toxic. It can be decreased with taking aspirin before niacin—this was discovered by Richard Kunin, MD, of San Francisco. The flushing is caused by the release of histamine, which dilates blood vessels. If you take niacin regularly, the flushing should diminish. Histamine is also released during allergic reactions, so niacin might alleviate the symptoms of some allergic reactions.

Sometimes, but not very often, very high doses of niacin may damage the liver, elevate blood sugar levels, and aggravate gout.

Q. What are the guidelines for taking niacin to lower cholesterol?

A. Abram Hoffer, MD, PhD, discovered the cholesterol-lowering effect of niacin in the 1950s. It works, and it's even approved by the Food and Drug Administration. But other physicians have modified Hoffer's original recommendations. Andrew Weil, MD, has suggested six rules for taking a therapeutic niacin regimen. Rule number one tells us to use only the inositol hexanicotinate form. Rule number two says that we should not use the time-release products because they are more likely to cause adverse reactions. Rule number three tells us not to exceed 1,000 mg at any one dose and not to take more than one capsule every eight hours. Rule number four is to have liver function tests prior to niacin therapy and at regular intervals while on the program, and to stop the niacin supplementation immediately if there is any elevation in the liver enzymes. (Elevated liver enzymes are often indicative of liver disease.) Stopping the niacin will usually cause the liver function to return to normal in a short time. Rule number five says to stop the niacin if you develop any gastrointestinal symptoms, and number six states that the serum cholesterol levels should be monitored at monthly intervals.

5.

Pantothenic Acid

Pantothenic acid is a component of one of the most important substances in your body, coenzyme A. Before any sugar can be burned for fuel, it must be converted to acetyl coenzyme A. Pantothenic acid is required for this conversion and for that reason, without it, you could not produce any substantial amount of energy.

Q. Is it hard to become severely deficient in pantothenic acid?

A. Probably not. The prefix *pan* in Greek means *everywhere*. Many natural foods contain moderate amounts of pantothenic acid. Good sources of pantothenic acid include all varieties of meats (beef, pork, chicken, fish), whole grains, brewer's yeast, legumes (peas, beans, peanuts, soybean), eggs, and cabbage vegetables (broccoli, cauliflower, Brussels sprouts). Still, there may be many situations in which you need extra amounts of it.

Q. What are some other reasons why we need pantothenic acid?

A. Pantothenic acid influences the way other vitamins do their jobs, and it is involved in the production of antibodies that fight microbes and cancer. It's also part of the chain of reactions that manufacture neurotransmitters and is needed for the production of the adrenal stress hormones. That is why it is called the anti-stress vitamin. It also helps convert food into energy and promotes the healing of wounds.

Q. What are the symptoms of a pantothenic acid deficiency?

A. People who lack adequate levels of pantothenic acid have "pins and needles" in their hands and feet, are tired, have headaches, and often have nausea.

Q. When I'm stressed, I tend to develop viral infections. Can pantothenic acid help?

A. I have seen many stressed-out patients who developed tension-related herpes infections (e.g., Epstein-Barr virus, shingles, oral and genital herpes). Most people carry herpes viruses and usually don't have outbreaks of the pain and sores unless they are under severe situational stress. In my experience, they usually improve very quickly on pantothenic acid therapy. In many people with long-term drug-resistant shingles, 2,000 mg of pantothenic acid each day for one week resolves the condition. Patients with herpes infections who are on a daily dose of 500 mg of pantothenic acid have very few exacerbations.

Whenever you are fighting a herpes infection, be it shingles or genital herpes, stay away from foods that are rich in the amino acid arginine. Peanuts, chocolate, nuts, peas, and other bean relatives have high levels of arginine. This food substance is important for the replication of the herpes viruses.

Q. I've heard that pantothenic acid can help my allergic rhinitis. Is that true?

A. It might be worth a try. One doctor wrote to the *Townsend Letter for Doctors* and reported that 250 mg of pantothenic acid twice a day reduced the symptoms of allergic rhinitis.

Q. Can pantothenic acid increase my immunity against many virus infections?

A. Yes. As Richard Huemer, MD, and Jack Challem

wrote in their book, *The Natural Health Guide to Beating the Supergerms* (Pocket Books, 1997), pantothenic acid is essential for the health of the thymus gland and antibody production. Antibodies attach themselves to viruses and identify them as alien, so the cells of the immune system can destroy them.

Q. Is it necessary to take other vitamins when I take pantothenic acid?

A. Yes, there are complicated interactions between many of the vitamins, especially the B group. If you are taking therapeutic amounts of any one B vitamin, you should also take a B-complex supplement for proper balance.

Q. My grandmother frequently has cold sores around her mouth—could this be a result of pantothenic acid deficiency?

A. Yes, it could. Many people in nursing homes are under both emotional and physical stress. Stress results in the activation and reproduction of various herpes viruses (cold sore viruses). During these periods, a person requires additional doses of pantothenic acid to help the immune system destroy the virus particles. In studies on the dietary intake of pantothenic acid among nursing homes residents, it was found that these people have much lower levels of pantothenic acid than the general population.

Q. I've heard about some people taking pantothenic acid during the winter. Why do they do that?

A. Exposure to cold increases the synthesis of coenzyme A, needed for energy and heat production in your cells. Pantothenic acid is required for the production of coenzyme A. So, in cold weather there is an increased consumption of pantothenic acid by your cells. As a result, it is possible to develop a pantothenic acid deficiency and consequently become susceptible to viral infections, such as colds and the flu.

Q. Can pantothenic acid help speed the healing of cuts?

A. Yes, I think so. I often prescribe doses of pantothenic acid and vitamin C to aid in the healing process. Several studies have shown that these vitamins improve the healing of skin lesions.

Q. Is there any disease state that would prohibit the use of pantothenic acid supplementation?

A. I would not take extra pantothenic acid supplementation if I had malaria because the malaria parasite requires high amounts of pantothenic in order to complete its life cycle.

Q. Is pantothenic acid helpful for heart disease?

A. Michael Murray, ND, and Joseph Pizzorno, ND, in their informative book *Encyclopedia of Natural Healing* (Prima Publishing, 1998) recommend pantothenic acid along with carnitine and coenzyme Q_{10} for heart disease patients because these supplements prevent the accumulation of fatty acids within the heart muscle. I have prescribed this combination along with alpha-lipoic acid and magnesium to my patients and have seen remarkable results.

Q. What is the RDA for pantothenic acid?

A. For adults, the RDA is about 4 to 10 mg a day. I personally take 500 mg a day when I am feeling good and take more when I feel a virus infection coming on.

6.

Vitamin B$_6$ and Folic Acid

___

Vitamin B$_6$ (pyridoxine) is necessary for the metabolism of amino acids, the building blocks of proteins, and the synthesis of neurotransmitters. Folic acid, which is required in very small amounts, is needed to repair DNA, which reduces genetic damage and the risk of cancer. These two vitamins work together to maintain low levels of homocysteine, a byproduct of protein metabolism associated with cardiovascular diseases.

Q. What are the signs and symptoms of vitamin B$_6$ deficiency?

___

A. Fatigue, anemia, gastrointestinal distress, elevated blood lipids, slow wound healing, inflammation of the tongue and mouth, and neurological symptoms such as seizures and pins and needles are some of the conditions that a person with a vitamin B_6 deficiency may exhibit.

Q. What foods contain large amounts of vitamin B_6?

A. Large amounts of this vitamin can be found in chicken, beef, fish, eggs, spinach, carrots, avocado, bananas, certain nuts, alfalfa, and whole wheat. Fresh foods, of course, contain higher levels of this and other vitamins compared with highly processed and overcooked foods.

Q. Can taking too much vitamin B_6 be toxic?

A. Pyridoxine in doses of hundreds of milligrams daily over several months has sometimes been found to cause loss of muscle coordination and nerve damage. I would not take more than 100 mg in any one single dose, and if I took any more that day, it would be at least eight hours later. If you feel you need more vitamin B_6, it would be prudent to get the advice of a doctor who understands vitamin physiology.

Q. Could vitamin B_6 help with acne?

A. Possibly yes. Acne vulgaris in adult women, in many cases, appears to be associated with a change in the balance between the female and male hormones. All of us produce some female and some male hormones, but stressful situations can upset their balance. Many naturopathic doctors believe that supplementation with pyridoxine can correct the balance.

Pyridoxine is also depleted through the normal metabolism of the sex hormones. So women of childbearing age, those who take birth control pills, and women who have had multiple pregnancies have an increased risk for the development of a pyridoxine deficiency. In men, scientists have reported that a low pyridoxine level results in a "using up" of testosterone.

So, getting back to the question, it may be possible to balance your sex hormones with vitamin supplementation, and you may be able to prevent some cases of acne. But I would not try this approach without first consulting a doctor who understands the manipulation of hormones with natural substances.

Q. Could vitamin B₆ help migraine headaches?

A. Again, probably. A migraine headache is the

result of the temporary dilation and excessive pulsation of the blood vessels leading to the brain. Stress, food allergies, food intolerance, flashing lights, and hormonal changes can bring on this condition. Many studies have shown that just by removing the offending foods from your diet, you can reduce the incidence of migraine from 40 to 70 percent. Wheat products, cow's milk, chocolate, beer, cheese, red wine, citrus fruit, and eggs are some of the common foods that trigger the events that lead to the headache. These foods contain histamine or increase the amount of histamine in your blood stream. These substances travel to blood vessels leading to your brain and cause the migraine.

There is an enzyme that breaks down histamine, and pyridoxine is necessary for its activity. So, if you avoid foods that cause headaches, reduce stress, and supplement your diet with reasonable doses of pyridoxine and riboflavin, you should be able to avoid most migraine headaches. Once more, each person is different, so a good natural or integrative doctor will help you set up an anti-migraine program.

Q. How important is vitamin B$_6$ prenatally?

A. It's very important, just as are folic acid and all the other B vitamins. Newborn animals whose mothers were very low in pyridoxine developed seizures and movement disorders. Likewise, newborn human infants who are deficient in pyridoxine may develop neurological symptoms. In addition, vitamin B$_6$ deficiency in pregnant women is associated with cleft palates in their offspring. It's important that all women of child-bearing age take a prenatal supplement, or multivitamin, that includes the B complex.

Q. Does vitamin B$_6$ really help with carpal tunnel syndrome?

A. Secretaries, assembly-line workers, supermarket cashiers, and others who type or do work that involves repetitive motion of the hands frequently develop carpal tunnel syndrome. Many years ago, John Ellis, MD, discovered that patients with carpal tunnel had low pyridoxine levels. He gave them 100 mg of pyridoxine a day for three months, which relieved the symptoms of the majority of patients. Bear in mind that people are rarely deficient in just one nutrient. I think 100 mg of vitamin B$_6$, plus a high-potency B-complex supplement, would be better than B$_6$ alone.

Q. Can nightly doses of vitamin B$_6$ help me sleep better?

A. In certain cases, yes. Some doctors believe that pyridoxine stimulates the pineal gland to secrete increased amounts of melatonin, and this helps a person get better sleep. One sign of inadequate vitamin B$_6$ is the inability to dream or recall dreams. Too much B$_6$ might give you dreams so vivid that you'll feel tired in the morning.

Q. Can vitamin B$_6$ help with asthma?

A. Many people with asthmatic conditions have difficulty metabolizing the amino acid tryptophan. Tryptophan can be changed into the neurotransmitter serotonin. Many doctors believe that high levels of serotonin can cause squeezing of the airways. High blood levels of the breakdown products of serotonin have been associated with severe asthma. Pyridoxine supplementation corrects the biochemical problems that many asthmatic people have with the metabolism of tryptophan, and, consequently, this therapy may improve their asthmatic condition.

Also, very high doses of the asthma drug theophylline may produce drug-induced seizures because it depletes pyridoxine. Veterinarians have used pyridoxine to reverse seizures from theophylline overdoses in animals for years. Using pyridoxine may also help people avoid theophylline-induced seizures.

Q. Can vitamin B₆ lower blood pressure?

A. It can. In Turkey, doctors gave twenty high blood pressure patients pyridoxine daily for four weeks. At the end of the study, most of the patients had significant drops in both their systolic (high number) and diastolic (low number) blood pressures.

Q. Does vitamin B₆ help AIDS?

A. Yes. HIV-infected and other immune-suppressed individuals often have low levels of pyridoxine. This vitamin is required for the normal operation of the immune system. It helps stimulate the immune response, and it helps activate the synthesis of antibodies. People with very low pyridoxine levels have a lower number of white blood cells that destroy disease organisms and that kill and eat cancer cells. In addition, scientists have found that people with pyridoxine deficiencies have poor thymus function. The thymus is the organ where many of the immune system cells are programmed to do their jobs.

Q. Is there any research on the suppression of cancer cells with vitamin B₆?

A. Yes. Vitamin B_6 stops the growth of liver cancer cells when added to tissue culture. Many women with cervical dysplasia or cancer of the cervix have low blood levels of B_6 levels. We know that pyridoxine is an essential substance for immunity against cancer, and we also know that this vitamin is involved with the metabolism of the female sex hormones. I think it would be interesting to study the preventative and healing potential of pyridoxine on estrogen-related cancers.

Q. In the Introduction, you described the use of pyridoxine for mushroom poisoning. Why is B₆ effective as an antidote?

A. Mushrooms are a breeding ground for fungi, and they are veritable toxin factories. Mushroom fungi live underground and are the largest living organisms yet found. The body (mycelium) of one individual fungus may grow through more than ten acres of soil and live for hundreds of years or more.

Pyridoxine is an antidote for *Gyromitra* mushroom poisoning. This fungus produces a water-soluble toxin that is identical in structure to certain rocket fuels and can cause a rapid illness that can result in death. Lower doses of *Gyromitra* toxins can cause a slow illness that can result in cancer. The *Gyromitra* toxin interferes with the metabolic production of pyridoxine and causes seizures, vomiting, cramps, diarrhea, liver destruction, and tumor formation, among other symptoms. Although fairly common, most cases of *Gyromitra* poisoning are misdiagnosed, and about 15 percent of people who eat *Gyromitra* mushrooms die. Chefs that cook *Gyromitra* mushrooms may also get sick from inhaling the fumes of this mushroom. If this illness is diagnosed properly, intravenous pyridoxine is life-saving.

Q. What is a good supplemental dose of vitamin B₆?

A. Very high doses of vitamin B₆—for example, more than 500 mg daily—for months can result in nerve damage. In general, I find it rare for a person to need more than 100 mg of B₆ daily, and most people do quite well with 10 to 25 mg daily as part of a B-complex supplement. If you want to take higher doses to treat a specific condition, such as carpal tunnel syndrome, please work with a physician.

"More" may not always be better; it may also be more expensive than a lower and equally effective dose.

Q. How do B$_6$ and folic acid affect homocysteine and heart disease?

A. Homocysteine is a toxic breakdown product of methionine, an essential component of protein. It damages blood vessel walls and sets the stage for cholesterol deposits. Homocysteine levels increase when the diet contains too little vitamin B$_6$ and folic acid relative to the amount of methionine (found in meat). Today, homocysteine is regarded as a cardio-vascular risk factor equal to, or more serious than, high cholesterol. Vitamin B$_6$ and folic acid play key roles in controlling homocysteine. So do vitamin B$_{12}$ and choline.

Q. What are some of the specific functions of folic acid?

A. Folic acid is necessary for the synthesis, utiliza-tion, and breakdown of amino acids and proteins. This B vitamin is also important for the synthesis and maintenance of the nucleic acids (DNA and RNA). Folic acid is an active participant in the production of the red blood cells that carry oxygen to all of our cells.

Q. What are the best dietary sources of folic acid?

A. It is found in leafy green vegetables, such as leaf lettuce and spinach, beet greens, asparagus, liver, kidney, oranges, pineapple, cantaloupe, bananas, lima beans, green peas, bean sprouts, whole wheat, and soybeans. Folic acid is very sensitive to heat, light, cooking, or even long-term storage at room temperature. When foods are processed, much of the folic acid is lost.

Q. Can a deficiency in folic acid lead to anemia?

A. Yes, and in addition to anemia (low red blood cell count), it can lead to problems with white blood cell function and poor antibody production. And these conditions can bring about a lack of immune activity and allow bacteria, viruses, fungi, and cancer cells to damage your body and cause serious diseases.

Q. What types of people must be certain that they get enough folic acid?

A. People who take prescription drugs, people with blood vessel disease, pregnant women, alcoholics, women on birth control pills, and people taking antibiotics that kill the bacteria in the intestines, must obtain enough folic acid, or they may suffer serious health problems.

Q. What are some signs of a folic acid deficiency?

A. Megaloblastic anemia (low numbers of red blood cells that are distended), low white cell counts, and sores in the gastrointestinal tract are common signs of a folic acid deficiency. Folic acid has had a lot of press related to pregnant women recently because it has been found that many women who gave birth to babies with neural-tube defects (e.g., spina bifida), are deficient in folic acid.

Q. I recent had an abnormal Pap smear (cervical dysplasia). Could folic acid help?

A. Probably, yes. Cervical dysplasia is frequently caused by one of the human papiloma viruses (wart viruses), is a sexually transmitted disease, and is considered by many to be precancerous. Tori

Hudson, ND, of Portland, Oregon, has seen very excellent results in treating cervical dysplasia with folic acid and a combination of other vitamins. She actually inserts vitamin suppositories into the cervix in order to put these healing nutrients in contact with the virus infection.

If the dysplasia is high grade it should be promptly treated with surgical technique; however, if your doctor tells you that it is low grade, you may have other choices. Many forms of viral dysplasia will clear up on their own in a few months. Other forms will progress to cervical cancer. With low-grade cervical dysplasias, folic acid supplementation, pyridoxine, beta-carotene, vitamin A, and certain other natural treatments have a high cure rate and are easier on your body than surgery. See your integrative or naturopathic doctor prior to starting on a nutritional program for cervical dysplasia.

Q. Can a severe deficiency in folic acid cause cancer?

A. Yes, I think so. Folic acid is necessary for the production and repair of your DNA. Damage to DNA is called a mutation, and a mutation may force a cell to develop into a cancer cell. Consequently, a deficiency in folic acid may lead to irreparable DNA mutations, and this condition may lead to cancer. I know some people who take extra folic acid and vitamin B_{12} to minimize their DNA damage from cancer, familial hyperlipidemia, and cystic fibrosis. One study shows that the combination does in fact reduce genetic damage.

Q. What is a good dose of folic acid?

A. Folic acid is exceptionally safe, and a daily dose of 400 to 800 mcg will lower homocysteine levels and presumably reduce the risk of cardiovascular disease. This dose will also reduce the risk of neural-tube defects in babies, though the mother must start taking the vitamin within the first couple weeks of pregnancy—or be taking it before getting pregnant.

The only major concern about folic acid is that it may mask the symptoms of a vitamin B_{12} deficiency. This masking issue does not usually become a problem unless a person takes more than 5,000 mcg (5 mg) of folic acid daily for an extended period of time. It's easily avoided by also taking a small amount of vitamin B_{12}. Because these two vitamins work together, as do all of the B vitamins, it's probably wiser to take the entire B complex as a single supplement.

7.

Vitamin B$_{12}$

Vitamin B$_{12}$ is a very large and complex molecule built around an atom of cobalt. The
secretion of a stomach chemical called "intrinsic
factor" governs the absorption of vitamin B$_{12}$.
Intrinsic factor combines with vitamin B$_{12}$ and
facilitates its passage through the wall of the
small intestine and into the blood stream. Vitamin
B$_{12}$ occurs in at least four forms in humans:
cyanocobalamin, methylcobalamin, hydroxycobal-
amin and adenosylcobalamin.

Q. Why is vitamin B$_{12}$ so important for good health?

A. It is required for the manufacture of the nucleic acids that make up genes, and the production of
energy from sugars and fats. It is also fundamental
to the formation of red blood cells. Vitamin B$_{12}$ is
necessary for the normal growth of the nervous system and the prevention of infertility. It also is need-

ed to produce the neurotransmitter acetylcholine, which is based on another B vitamin, choline.

Q. I am a strict vegetarian, do I need B_{12} supplements?

A. Yes. Vitamin B_{12} is found only in foods of animal origin. Milk, cheese, fish, or meat are considered to be the only important sources of this vitamin. Organ meats such as liver are the best sources of vitamin B_{12}. So if you are a very strict vegetarian, such as a vegan, you may require some vitamin B_{12} supplementation.

Q. What are the symptoms of a vitamin B_{12} deficiency?

A. Fatigue, anemia, pale complexion, forgetfulness, pins-and-needles and numbness of the toes, and burning feet are common symptoms of a lack of vitamin B_{12}.

Q. What does vitamin B_{12} have to do with anemia?

A. If you don't obtain adequate quantities of vitamin B_{12}, you may become anemic because vitamin

B_{12} is required for the production of red blood cells. Some people's stomachs do not produce either sufficient hydrochloric acid or intrinsic factor. If a person does not have enough hydrochloric acid, intrinsic factor, and certain digestive enzymes, a person cannot absorb sufficient amounts of B_{12}. People who eat a lot of junk foods—potato chips, desserts, soft drinks—may develop severe fatigue and shortness of breath related to vitamin B_{12} deficiency anemia.

Q. Do older people require more vitamin B_{12} supplementation than young people?

A. Scientists have reported that vitamin B_{12} levels decline with age. This may be due to reduced intake, unhealthy diets, or poor absorption. Production of intrinsic factor does decline with age, and this will impair vitamin B_{12} absorption. Some studies have found that as many as one-third of people over age 65 suffer from atrophic gastritis—a long-term inflammation of the intestines, with a breakdown of intrinsic factor and acid-secreting cells—which will interfere with B_{12} absorption. Injections of B_{12} and sublingual (under the tongue) supplements should overcome this problem.

Q. I've heard that vitamin B_{12} is necessary for normal immunity. Is this true?

A. Yes, it is. Vitamin B_{12} deficiency may result in diminished white blood cell production and abnormal white blood cell behavior. These cells normally move through the tissues and travel around the blood stream in search of cancer cells and dangerous microbes. If they are not provided with adequate amounts of vitamin B_{12}, they cannot do their jobs.

Q. Why do so many people with AIDS take vitamin B_{12}?

A. Many people with AIDS have low B_{12} levels. This may occur as a result of decreased absorption, reduced ingestion, or antagonism by anti-viral drugs. It is also true that as AIDS progresses, blood levels of B_{12} fall further. This complicates things because B_{12} is indispensable for good immune function. In addition, vitamin B_{12} inhibits reproduction of the HIV virus in cell-culture studies, and it may hold promise as one of the standard future therapies for AIDS. So taking supplemental B_{12} is a good idea.

Q. Do people with Crohn's disease need more vitamin B$_{12}$?

A. They likely do. Crohn's disease is a painful inflammatory condition that may damage any part of the digestive tract. Most cases, however, occur in the mid-part of the small intestines. This disease may destroy the entire wall of the intestines sometimes even forming deep ulcers that evolve into penetrating holes. A healthy mid-intestine is necessary for B$_{12}$ absorption. So people with this inflammatory bowel condition are often vitamin B$_{12}$ deficient and require supplementation.

Q. How does vitamin B$_{12}$ affect fertility in men?

A. Vitamin B$_{12}$ is required for normal cell division in any cell and consequently it is especially necessary for the production of quickly dividing sperm cells. Men who have low vitamin B$_{12}$ levels often have low sperm counts and poor sperm motility. In addition, men with low sperm counts tend to be deficient in antioxidant vitamins, such as vitamins E and C.

Q. Can vitamin B$_{12}$ supplementation help multiple sclerosis?

A. Yes, in certain ways. People with MS suffer damage to the protective coverings of the nerve fibers, the myelin sheaths. The damage to the nerves results in paralysis or partial paralysis. Many microbiologists think the initial damage to the nerve sheath is caused by a herpesvirus and further damage is produced by the person's own over-active immune system.

Vitamin B$_{12}$ deficiencies also have been shown to cause similar damage to the myelin sheaths and many people with MS have low vitamin B$_{12}$ levels. Some scientists have reported that high doses of vitamin B$_{12}$ may increase brain function and improve eyesight in MS patients, but don't appear to reverse the paralysis. If you have MS, it would be best to get regular B$_{12}$ shots from your doctor to see if they help.

Q. Do you think that vitamin B$_{12}$ can improve my memory?

A. Many of my patients who receive this vitamin tell me that with B$_{12}$ they can think more effectively and have improved memory. It may not work the same way for everyone, but if you forget a lot of things, it's certainly worth a try. One study found that older people who were senile were deficient in B$_{12}$, and some of them became sharper with supplementation.

Q. Will vitamin B$_{12}$ help with dandruff?

A. There is a great amount of anecdotal information suggesting that B$_{12}$ is helpful in the treatment of many skin conditions, including dandruff and some forms of eczema. Some patients have had great success with B$_{12}$. This may be due to B$_{12}$'s involvement, along with choline, in the production of a beneficial skin substance called tetrahydrofolate.

Q. How much vitamin B$_{12}$ should a person take?

A. I think the officially recommended amount—2 mcg daily—is ridiculously low. Part of the problem is poor absorption and poor production of intrinsic factor, which controls B$_{12}$ absorption. These absorption-related problems increase with age, but they can be overcome at any age in a number of ways. The simplest is to take a sublingual B$_{12}$ tablet. Sublingual means it dissolves under the tongue. There is a network of blood vessels under the tongue that readily and directly absorb what is placed there. Taking B_{12} in this way bypasses the digestive system and the need for intrinsic factor. I think 100 to 500 mcg of vitamin B_{12} is a reasonable dosage. Excesses are harmless and excreted.

8.

Choline and Inositol

In 1998, choline was finally classified as an essential B vitamin. It forms the core of a key neurotransmitter acetylcholine, which is needed for thinking processes. Inositol is a B vitamin involved in the health of cell membranes, liver function, and normal immunity.

Q. What are some good sources of choline?

A. Eggs and soybeans are rich sources of this nutrient. Every living cell contains choline, and lecithin contains a great amount of it. Lecithin plays an important role in cell membrane function, nerve cell performance, and fat metabolism. Choline can also be synthesized by the normal flora bacteria in your intestines and absorbed into your blood stream. Cooking may destroy the choline in foods.

Q. What does the term emulsification mean, and what does it have to do with choline?

A. Emulsification is the production of a watery liquid from a suspension of fat molecules. During emulsification, the surface tension of water is lowered and fats can be dissolved. This process is necessary for the absorption of fats by the intestinal wall.

Choline is a component of phosphatidylcholine molecule, and phosphatidylcholine is a part of the lecithin molecule. Lecithin is the primary emulsification agent in bile and is responsible for the proper absorption of cholesterol, fats, vitamins A, D, E, K, and thiamin. The food industry often adds lecithin in order to keep fats in a soluble state.

Q. What are the symptoms of choline deficiency?

A. A severe choline deficiency would cause death. Without choline, all cell membranes would fall apart, and the body would cease to function.

Q. Is it safe to give choline to pregnant women and young babies?

A. Yes, and it may even help brain function in babies. One study found that giving choline to young animals improves their memory and task performance.

Q. How is choline involved in brain development?

A. Acetylcholine is a key neurotransmitter that is synthesized from choline and acetic acid. Your brain can't work without it, and your body cannot make acetylcholine without choline. Scientific studies have shown that inadequate levels of choline in developing brains result in increased cell death. Therefore, you need adequate choline for normal brain development.

Q. I've heard that *Ginkgo biloba* can protect the brain—does this have anything to do with choline?

A. Under conditions of low oxygen tension, as with strokes, brain cell membranes are disrupted and choline leaks out into the intercellular fluid. *Ginkgo biloba* extract has been reported to curb disruption of the cell membranes and help choline in brain cells.

Q. Will choline help prevent Alzheimer's disease?

A. The evidence so far has been mixed. It seems to help some patients, but not others. The reason is probably related to the complicated nature of Alzheimer's disease. Some neurologists think that the leakage of choline from brain cells results in the development of Alzheimer's disease. Beta-amyloid protein is found in the brains of Alzheimer's disease patients. As increased amounts of beta-amyloid are laid down, more choline is squeezed out of the cell. This leads to a reduction of neurotransmitters and consequently a decline in brain function. I would not depend solely on choline to reduce the risk of Alzheimer's disease. I would, at the very least, combine it with vitamin B_{12} and carnitine.

Q. Why do some doctors give choline supplements to people with asthma?

A. Asthma is an inflammatory disease that involves the lungs and its air tubes. Choline has some very powerful anti-inflammatory properties. Studies were done to compare the effectiveness of choline supplementation with a well-known prescription drug in people of various ages. Choline was found to be at least as effective as the prescription drug for asthma prevention. Furthermore, a dose of 1,000 mg was found to be more effective than a dose of 500 mg of choline. An added benefit is that side effects from choline are very rare.

Q. How is choline involved in liver health?

A. It's involved in two major ways. As an emulsifier, choline is thought to be helpful in dissolving some of the fat stored in the liver. When a person with a damaged fatty liver is given oral choline, the fat content has been demonstrated to fall. In addition, it has also been shown that a choline-deficient diet can induce the development of liver cancer in some animals. Moreover, when liver cells are grown in 9 culture and deprived of choline, the normal programmed death of cells is altered. Normal cells live to a certain age and then commit "cell suicide." Cancer cells just keep growing and don't know how to die properly. Some researchers think that a deficiency of choline may interfere with the normal life and death cycles and can lead to the development of cancer.

Q. What are the symptoms of inositol deficiency?

A. Naturally occurring inositol deficiency in humans has never been found. In mice, a lack of inositol results in visual defects, neurological disease, loss of hair, and growth failure. Although it is difficult to know how animal studies relate to human lives, an inositol deficiency in humans would probably lead to the same conditions.

Q. What are some good dietary sources of inositol?

A. Inositol can be found in sufficient amounts in whole grains, fruits, meat, dairy products, and yeast cells.

Q. Is it true that alcohol abuse can lead to a severe inositol deficiency and result in brain disease?

A. This is true. Many chemical messengers in the brain require inositol-containing substances in order to operate. Large quantities of alcohol interfere with the production of these substances and consequently may lead to memory, behavior, and other mental problems.

Q. What are some medical uses of inositol?

A. Some doctors use this vitamin to help lower cholesterol levels, help restore injured skin, prevent hardening of the arteries, and protect the heart.

Some of the most interesting recent developments relate to its use in treating psychiatric disorders. Doctors have found that high doses of inositol are very effective in reducing depression, panic attacks, and obsessive-compulsive behavior. The effective dose for these conditions seems to range from about 12 to 18 gm daily.

Q. What is signal transduction, and how is inositol involved in it?

A. Signal transduction is a normal process by which a chemical message is passed from the outer shell (membrane) of a cell and into the center of the cell (cell nucleus). A chemical messenger (cytokine) or other molecule binds to a cell membrane and causes a protein to undergo a chemical change in this membrane. Then the chemical message is passed down through the cell in a series of reactions until it ultimately reaches the nucleus. Inositol molecules combined with high-energy phosphorus-containing compounds are key players in this process.

Q. Can choline and inositol help with premenstrual syndrome (PMS)?

A. Years ago, Carlton Fredericks, PhD, recommended that women with high estrogen profiles take these two supplements. He contended that they help the liver break down estrogen into estriol, a safe and noncarcinogenic form of the hormone. Choline and inositol seem to work for many women with PMS. I would recommend taking supplements of these two B vitamins in addition to a regular B-complex supplement.

Q. I've been hearing about IP-6. What is it?

A. It is also called inositol hexaphosphate. Recent research using cell cultures and small animals have found that it may be helpful in preventing or treating cancer. Although promising, no human studies have so far been conducted. I might consider including it as part of a broader cancer-treatment program, but I would not use it by itself.

Q. How much choline and inositol should I take each day?

A. I think that with these vitamins, dosage should be custom tailored for a particular condition. If you have one of the conditions that may require inositol supplementation, you may eat foods rich in this vitamin, or see a health professional who understands the physiology of this substance, and he could suggest a proper supplement dose. In general, though, many supplements contain 250 mg each of choline and inositol, and this appears to be a safe amount.

9.

Biotin and PABA

Biotin and para-amino benzoic acid (PABA) are two little known B vitamins. Although they don't have a lot of pizzazz, compared with other vitamins, they are still important for health.

Q. Why is biotin so important for good health?

A. Biotin is needed by the body to break down fats and to create new ones. It also plays an important role in the construction of proteins from amino acids and helps manufacture certain building blocks of genes. In addition, biotin is necessary for the normal development of white blood cells that fight germs and destroy cancer cells. Low biotin levels may result in the weakening of your immune system.

Q. What are the symptoms of biotin deficiency?

A. People who are low in biotin may be anemic and pale, have poor appetites, and may have muscle pains, flaking of their skin, "pins and needles" in their toes, and a feeling of soreness in their tongues.

Q. I heard that eating too many eggs could make you biotin deficient. Is that true?

A. This is a problem with only raw egg whites. People who eat a lot of raw eggs may develop a biotin deficiency. Avidin, a chemical in raw egg white, combines with biotin and forms a substance that is excreted from the body. All cells require biotin to stay alive. Normal cells cannot use the biotin if it is bound chemically to avidin. Cooking destroys avidin.

Q. Do older people often develop biotin deficiencies?

A. They might. Japanese scientists asked this same question and studied several hundred people over 65 years old. Some of the participants had normal biotin levels and some had very low biotin levels. The scientists concluded that the blood biotin levels of senior citizens vary greatly. Part of the problem is that the efficiency of absorption declines with age. This makes eating a high-quality diet and taking supplements particularly important as you age.

Q. What foods contain large amounts of biotin?

A. Biotin is found in most natural foods in relatively small amounts. Greater amounts of biotin are found in organ meats, egg yolks, fungal products such as brewer's yeast, natural whole grains, and milk products. Normally, the bacteria in our digestive tracts produce sufficient quantities of biotin.

Q. I've heard that vegetarians have the lowest rates of biotin deficiency. Why?

A. Vegetarians usually have very large healthy colonies of bacteria in their colon. This is partly because vegetarians tend to eat a lot of fermented foods, rich in beneficial bacteria. These bacteria are responsible for producing appreciable amounts of biotin.

If you take antibiotics several times a year, it might be wise to supplement with about 400 mcg of biotin daily. Many beneficial bacteria are killed when a person takes oral antibiotics. While antibiotics can curb bacterial infections, they disrupt digestion. In addition, taking acidophilus capsules can help restore normal intestinal bacteria.

Q. Can biotin help in diabetes?

A. It can help in adult-onset, or Type II, diabetes. Scientists have demonstrated that biotin supplementation can increase the cell's sensitivity to insulin so it can utilize glucose more efficiently.

Q. What are some general functions of PABA?

A. PABA is required for a metabolic cycle termed the "tetrahydrofolate acid cycle." This series of biochemical reactions assists in the metabolism of amino acids. PABA also functions in the formation of blood cells. PABA is found in organ meats, such as liver, as well as in wheat germ, whole grains, eggs, and brewer's yeast.

Q. What are some medical uses for PABA?

A. PABA appears to be a good sunscreen because it shields the skin from ultraviolet light. Some information exists that it may be useful for osteoarthritis, skin revitalization, and for reversing gray hair. I have not personally seen it work for these conditions. In very high doses, PABA may cause some damage to the liver. Some people have also reported nausea and vomiting and allergic-type symptoms.

Q. Can PABA diminish the effectiveness of sulfa antibiotics?

A. Very large amounts could. There are many disease-causing bacteria that require PABA as a building block for the synthesis of folic acid. Folic acid is necessary for other vitamin synthesis and amino acid formation. The sulfa drug molecule is very similar in structure to the PABA molecule. Because of this, certain bacteria are confused, and use the sulfa drug in place of the PABA molecule. In this way, in bacteria, sulfa drugs interfere with the formation of the needed vitamin folic acid. It is thought that if a great amount of PABA is available during sulfa drug treatment, this vitamin will interfere with the effectiveness of the antibiotic. Conversely, I believe that following long-term sulfa drug adminstration, it might be wise to supplement with PABA.

Q. How much biotin and PABA should a person take?

A. There are not many circumstances in which a person will have to take very large doses of just biotin and PABA. For this reason, I recommend that you take what comes in a B-complex supplement. Of course, a health professional who knows your medical history may recommend high doses for you, and this is perfectly all right.

Conclusion

Perhaps overshadowed by antioxidants and other headline-making nutrients, the B-complex vitamins are fundamentally important to health. Many of the problems people suffer—physical and psychiatric problems—can be alleviated with the B vitamins. This is good medicine because it uses natural and safe substances to optimize health.

The B vitamins comprise a group of related nutrients needed for the normal operation of your immune system, nervous system, respiratory system, detoxification system, and every other system of your body. These actions might seem broad, but it is because the B vitamins are required by every cell in your body, and you would get sick and die without them. A deficiency in certain B vitamins could produce a condition in which serious damage to the nucleic acids, which are responsible for who you are and who you will become, is not repaired. This can result in cancer, altered genetics, or premature death.

I cannot give you a specific prescription for your daily doses of B vitamins because each person, depending on his or her medical condition, sex, weight, age, amount of physical and mental stress, and diet requires a specially customized B vitamin program. A knowledgeable integrative or naturo-pathic doctor can design such a program for you. Health-food stores and pharmacies contain an assortment of excellent B-complex supplements in various dosages, and their staff can help you select an appropriate one.

I personally take two high quality B-complex capsules every day, one with each meal. To that I add 250 mg of extra pantothenic acid, 100 mg of alpha-lipoic acid, and coenzyme Q_{10}. I also take a good multi-vitamin, 400 IU of vitamin E, 25,000 IU of beta-carotene, and a 200 mcg capsule of natural selenium. I also make a point of eating a healthy diet with at least six servings of vegetables each day. I make sure that I get to the gym three days a week where I do sensible weight training and jog 1 to 2 miles a session. Since I've been on that program, I have felt great.

Glossary

Antibodies. Proteins produced by the immune system cells. Antibodies bind to the surfaces of invading substances and organisms.

Antioxidant. A chemical that obstructs, restrains, or neutralizes a product of oxidation.

Coenzyme. A molecule necessary for proper enzyme function.

Enzyme. A protein produced by the body that acts as a catalyst in chemical reactions.

Free radicals. Highly reactive atoms or molecules with one or more unpaired electrons.

Immune system. The organs, cells, and proteins that work together to protect the body from foreign substances. Includes the liver, spleen, thymus, bone marrow, and lymph system.

Neurotransmitter. A substance that passes chemical messages from one nerve cell to other cells.

Nucleic acids. The building blocks of proteins. Found in the fungal, animal, bacterial, and plant kingdoms.

Placebo. A capsule, pill, or injectable solution that does not contain a pharmacologically active substance.

Protein. A complex molecule made up of amino acid units. Proteins are responsible for building cell structures and controlling chemical reactions in the cells.

Stroke. A blockage of blood to the brain. If the blockage lasts for a period of time, it may cause destruction of brain tissue, which can result in paralysis, inability to talk, or death.

References

The information in this book is drawn from several hundred scientific references. These are some of those references.

Aybak M, et al., "Effect of oral pyridoxine hydrochloride supplementation on arterial blood pressure in patients with essential hypertension," *Arzneimittelforschung* 45 (1995): 1271–1273.

Berkson B, "Alpha-lipoic acid: My experience with this outstanding therapeutic agent," *Journal of Orthomolecular Medicine* 13 (1998): 44–48.

Gaur S, et al., "Use of LPC antagonist, choline, in the management of bronchial asthma," *Indian Journal of Chest Disease and Allied Science* 39 (1997): 107–113.

Jacobsson C and Granstrom G, "Effects of vitamin B_6 on beta-aminoproprionitrile-induced palatal cleft formation in the rat," *Cleft Palate Craniofacial Journal* 34 (1997): 95–100.

Kira S, et al., "Vitamin B$_{12}$ metabolism and massive-dose methyl vitamin B$_{12}$ therapy in Japanese patients with multiple sclerosis," *Internal Medicine* 33 (1994): 82–86.

Levine J, "Controlled trials of inositol in psychiatry," European *Neuropsychopharmacology* 7 (1997): 147–155.

Murray M and Srinivasan A, "Nicotinamide inhibits HIV-1 in both acute and chronic in vitro infection," *Biochemical and Biophysical Research Communications* 210 (1995): 954–959.

Schoenen J, et al., "Effectiveness of high-dose riboflavin in migraine prophylaxis. A randomized controlled trial," *Neurology* 50 (1998): 466–470.

Stone C, et al., "Effect of nicotinic acid on exogenous myocardial glucose utilization," *Journal of Nuclear Medicine* 36 (1995): 996–1002.

Walsh J, et al., "Pantothenic acid content of a nursing home diet," *Annals Nutrition Metabolism* 25 (1981): 178–181.

Webster R, et al., "Modulation of carcinogen-induced DNA damage and repair enzyme activity by dietary riboflavin," *Cancer Letter* 98 (1996): 129–135.

Suggested Readings

Balch JF and Balch PA. *Prescription for Nutritional Healing,* second edition. Garden City Park, NY: Avery Publishing Group, 1997.

Berkson B. *Alpha-Lipoic Acid Breakthrough.* Rocklin, CA: Prima Publishing, 1998.

Bock K and Sabin N. *The Road to Immunity.* New York: Pocket Books, 1997.

Huemer R and Challem J. *The Natural Health Guide to Beating the Supergerms.* New York: Pocket Books, 1997.

Murray M and Pizzorno J. *Encyclopedia of Natural Medicine.* Rocklin, CA: Prima Publishing, 1998.

Reuben C. *Antioxidants; Your Complete Guide.* Rocklin, CA: Prima Publishing, 1995.

Weil A. *Spontaneous Healing.* New York: Alfred A. Knopf, 1995.

Whitaker J. *Dr. Whitaker's Guide to Natural Healing.* Rocklin, CA: Prima Publishing, 1995.

Index

Acetyl coenzyme A, 43, 47

Acetylcholine, 73

Acne vulgaris, 51

Acquired immune deficiency
    syndrome, 40, 55, 66

AIDS. *See* Acquired immune
    deficiency syndrome.

Alzheimer's disease, 26–27, 74

Anemia, 60, 64–65

Antibiotics, effect on B vitamin
    levels, 12

Arginine, 45

Ariboflavinosis, 29–30

Asthma, 74–75

B-complex vitamins, 10, 13–17,
    53. *See also* B vitamins.

B vitamins
    antibiotics and, 12
    antioxidants, as, 14
    cooking's effect on, 13
    defined, 9–10
    dosage, recommended, 16–17
    sources of, 11
    U.S. recommended daily
        allowance of, 11–12
    See also B-complex vitamins;
        Biotin; Choline; Folic acid;
        Inositol; Niacin;

Niacinamide; PABA;
    Pantothenic acid;
    Pyridoxine; Riboflavin;
    Thiamin; Vitamin B$_{12}$;

Bell's palsy, 26

Beriberi, 12, 20

Biotin
    aging and, 82–83
    deficiency, 81–82
    diabetes and, 84
    dosage, recommended, 86
    importance of, 81
    sources of, 83

Blood pressure, 55

Cancer, 15, 31, 38, 56

Carpal tunnel syndrome, 53

Cervical dysplasia, 60–61

Cheilosis, 33

Cholesterol, 36–37, 41

Choline
    Alzheimer's disease and, 74
    asthma and, 74–75
    brain development and, 73
    deficiency, 72
    dosage, recommended, 79
    emulsification and, 72
    ginkgo biloba and, 73
    liver health and, 75

PMS and, 78
sources of, 71
Coenzyme A. *See* Acetyl coenzyme A.
Cyanocobalamin. *See* Vitamin B$_{12}$.
Diabetes, 27, 84
Folic acid
 cervical dysplasia and, 60–61
 deficiency, 59, 60
 DNA damage and, 61–62
 dosage, recommended, 62
 function of, 58–59
 heart disease and, 58
 homocysteine and, 58
 PABA and, 85
 sources of, 59
 vitamin B$_{12}$ deficiency and, 62
Gyromitra, 56–57
Headaches, 51–52
Heart disease, 14, 48, 58
Herpes infection, 45
Homocysteine, 14, 58
Infections, viral, 44–45
Inositol
 alcohol abuse and, 76
 deficiency, 75–76
 dosage, recommended, 79
 medical uses of, 77
 premenstrual syndrome and, 78
 signal transduction and, 77–78
 sources of, 76
Multiple sclerosis, 68
Niacin
 AIDS and, 40
 cancer and, 38

cholesterol levels and, 36–37, 41
 deficiency of, 39
 Raynaud's syndrome and, 37
 schizophrenia and, 37
 sources of , 36
 toxicity of, 40
 U.S. recommended daily allowance of, 35–36
Niacinamide
 AIDS and, 40
 schizophrenia and, 37
 U.S. recommended daily allowance of, 35–36
 See also Niacin.
Nicotinamide. *See* Niacinamide.
Nicotinamide adenine dinucleotide (NAD), 38, 39
Nicotinic acid. *See* Niacin.
PABA
 antibiotics and, 85
 dosage, recommended, 86
 function of, 84
 medical uses of, 84–85
Pantothenic acid
 Bell's palsy and, 26
 cold sores and, 46–47
 deficiency, 44
 function of, 44
 heart disease and, 48
 herpes and, 45
 infections, viral, and, 44–45
 infections, virus, and, 45–46
 malaria and, 48
 rhinitis and, 45
 sources of, 43
 U.S. recommended daily

allowance of, 48
vitamins, other, and, 46
Para-amino benzoic acid. *See*
PABA.
Pellagra, 12, 39
Premenstrual syndrome (PMS),
78
Pyridoxine
acne and, 51
AIDS and, 55
asthma and, 54–55
blood pressure and, 55
cancer and, 56
carpal tunnel syndrome and, 53
deficiency, 49–50
dosage, recommended, 57–58
gyromitra and, 57
headaches and, 51–52
heart disease and, 58
homocysteine and, 58
prenatal supplements of, 53
sleep and, 54
sources of, 50
toxicity of, 50
Raynaud's syndrome, 37
Rheumatoid arthritis, 31–32
Rhinitis, 45
Riboflavin
cancer and, 31
deficiency, 29–30, 33
dosage, recommended, 33
function of, 32
headaches and, 30–31
rheumatoid arthritis and, 31–32
sources of, 30
Schizophrenia, 37

Serotonin, 54
Stress, 15
Thiamin
aging and, 26
alcohol and, 23
Bell's palsy and, 26
deficiency, 20, 22, 23
depression and, 25
diabetes and, 27
effect on the body, 21
genetic diseases and, 23–24
smoking and, 22
sources of, 19–20
U.S. recommended daily
allowance, 24
Townsend Letter for Doctors, 45
Trytophan, 54
Vitamin B_1. *See* Thiamin.
Vitamin B_2. *See* Riboflavin.
Vitamin B_3. *See* Niacin;
Niacinamide.
Vitamin B_6. *See* Pyridoxine.
Vitamin B_{12}
aging and, 65
AIDS and, 66
anemia and, 64–65
Crohn's disease and, 67
deficiency, 62, 64
dosage, recommended, 69–70
fertility and, 67
immunity and, 66
importance of, 63–64
memory and, 68–69
multiple sclerosis, 68
skin conditions and, 69
vegetarians and, 64